Four Herbs for Health

Cooking with Herbs for Better Health

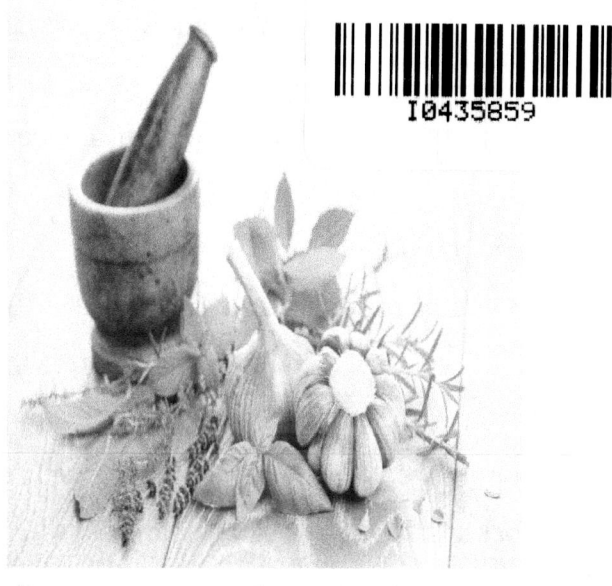

I0435859

By
Paolo Jose de Luna

Paolo Jose de Luna

unless with written permission from the publisher. All rights reserved.

The information provided herein is stated to be truthful and consistent, in that any liability, in terms of inattention or otherwise, by any usage or abuse of any policies, processes, or directions contained within is the solitary and utter responsibility of the recipient reader. Under no circumstances will any legal responsibility or blame be held against the publisher for any reparation, damages, or monetary loss due to the information herein, either directly or indirectly.

Respective authors own all copyrights not held by the publisher.

Table of Contents

Introduction

Herbs –the little leafy greens that we've all known and love. These little pieces of green goodness sure do pack a punch as herbs bear a variety of uses and they exhume an intense amount of flavor, possess a mix of wonderful fragrances, and have a number of benefits when it comes to our health.

Though they may be little in size, the greens that we call as "herbs" often pack a lot of power and finesse that boosts anyone's cooking any day. In the right hands and with the right ingredients, herbs can make outstanding dishes that radiate identity, fragrance, and deliciousness that no one in the world can match.

Herbs has a variety of uses, from perfumes up to medicine, herbs can bring magic into anything that you can think of. This versatility is what makes herbs so useful in our everyday lives that you can't possibly think of not having herbs around the house for everyday use.

Herbs in cooking isn't something new. A lot of dishes make use of these greens as a vibrant addition to plating and presentation. But even more dishes make use of herbs because of the fragrance and flavor that they add to the food. In fact, almost every high class restaurant has no main course dish that doesn't make use of herbs in one way or another because of all the things that it can do and enhance. Having herbs in your own kitchen is essential if you want to elevate your level of cooking.

Next up is fragrance as herbs aren't new to that either. Herbs enhance fragrance of countless perfumes and scents, giving a heightened level of smell with a wide variety of classes. One of the most common uses of herbs in potpourri as they can be made into oils and oil extracts and be used as potpourri scents that make your whole house smell majestic and sweet.

Aside from those, herbs can also be used in a variety of traditions and cultures, with some being regarded as "sacred herbs" because of their role in religious practices. Herbs like myrrh, turmeric, and cannabis bear an important meaning for a number of religions which are valued by worshippers.

Lastly, herbs become the lifeblood of herbal medicine. In fact, herbs are considered as a very important source of medicine as the sophisticated tools and methods in creating medicines didn't exist back then. Years ago, herbs were crushed and mixed together to create potions, teas, tonics, and remedies that serve as cures to a variety of diseases. You may call it a hoax, but the evidence in traditional medicine has proven that the use of herbs in early medicine has put forth a number of innovations that tell us that herbs have a lot of benefits towards our health.

Though herbs have a variety of powerful uses, you can easily get them in the supermarket or you can even grow them in your own garden. It's not that hard to obtain herbs, but most people tend to overlook the benefits that herbs have to offer and make a pass at them. If you think otherwise and want to explore more on the benefits of herbs, then this book is the right thing for you.

In this book, you'll be learning the best herbs that you can get your hands on and how these herbs can promote your health overall. You'll get to know everything about these herbs, including their backgrounds, their uses, how to get them, how to grow them, their benefits towards your health, and even how to use them in some of your cooking. You'd be amazed at how these seven essential herbs that you can find in the kitchen can spice things up for a variety of dishes and still boost your health in a number of ways that you might not even imagine.

Chapter 1 - All About Rosemary

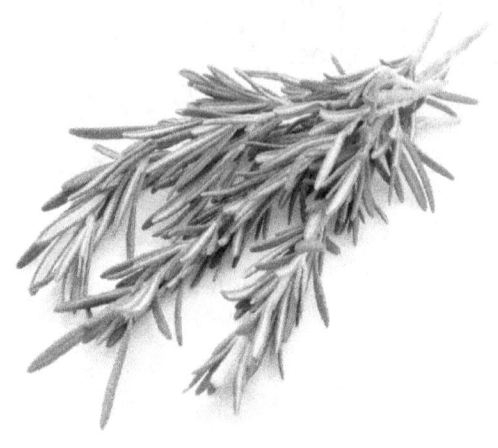

Officially known as *Rosmarinusofficinalis*, rosemary is a perennial herb characterized for its wooden body, its fragrant green leaves, and its flowers that may come in either pink, white, blue, or purple. Rosemary grows natively around the Mediterranean region, making it a staple herb among the countries located in Europe. Because of its rich fibrous root system, rosemary is considered to be one of the most unique herbs in the world. Rosemary belongs to the *Maliaceae* family of mints which include a variety of other herbs. At times, rosemary is also called *Anthos*, coming from the ancient Greek roots of its use which means "flower".

Characteristics

Rosemary is known as an aromatic and fragrant evergreen shrub that more or less looks very analogous to hemlock needles. It can grow upright or even trailing. Upright rosemary herbs can grow as tall as 5 feet, but they can rarely grow as tall as 6 feet to 7 feet. The evergreen leaves of this perennial herb can grow as much as 2 to 4 cm and these leaves have a 2 to 5 mm woolly hair – dense and short in shape – that's green above the leaves and white below the leaves.

The flowers of the rosemary often grow during the spring and summer when they're grown in temperate climates. However, the flowers can be found in full bloom throughout the seasons when they're grown in warmer climates. The rosemary's flowers can be found as pink, white, purple, or blue which brings a vibrant addition to any garden. Furthermore, the flowers can bloom without following the usual flowering season, blooming during the early December up to the middle of February.

Use of Rosemary in Cooking

Whether dried or fresh, rosemary can be used in a variety of dishes. Since rosemary is native to the Mediterranean region, the herb is never absent from most Italian cuisines.

Because of its tangy and bitter taste and its rich aroma, it complements most of the Italian dishes that are rich in tomatoes, cheeses, and wines. This herb also works well with pizza, tomato sauce, turkey, pasta, and grilled meat.

Rosemary is often partnered with a variety of meats and vegetables, adding fragrance and flavor. The mustard-like fragrance of rosemary when it's roasted is perfect to go with friend or barbecued dishes. Rosemary goes well with roasted meat, garlic, olive oil, and eggs. But because of its strong flavor and aroma, you need to be gentle in handling rosemary herbs because it can lose its flavor and fragrance if you don't handle it properly.

Because it is usually used to add flavor and aroma to food, rosemary is only used in a very small amount, thus bearing little nutritional benefits. But that doesn't mean that rosemary doesn't have benefits towards your health.

If you want to store rosemary in your kitchen pantry properly, you need to store it where you can provide it with moisture to keep it fresh and aromatic.

Health Benefits of Rosemary

While small in size, the rosemary sure does pack quite the punch. Possessing a strong flavor and aromatic scent, this herb is more than what it looks. Aside from being known as a staple herb ingredient in the kitchen for a number of dishes, it's also known to possess a number of benefits towards our health. Here are a few of the health benefits that you can get from rosemary.

- **Rich Anti-Oxidant** – Free radicals are harmful substances found in all sorts of places – food, chemicals, environment – almost everything can contain free radicals. These damage the cells and cripple the immune system, affecting your health. The only way to combat these free radicals is through anti-oxidants which can be found plenty in rosemary, as well as other foods.

- **Promote Skin Health** – The skin is the largest organ of the body and it's exposed to damage quite often. With pollution, heat, and germs, the skin sustains damage throughout the day. Rosemary is rich in anti-oxidants which help in preventing damage from free radicals that come from these factors, protecting the skin and promoting the growth of newer and healthier skin cells, giving you smoother skin.

- **Relieves Indigestion** – Rosemary helps by promoting gastric and intestinal motility and relieving dyspepsia. If you're feeling bloated and excessively full, trying taking a rosemary-based oil or even including some rosemary into your dishes and you'll feel quite the relief from all that gas built up in your stomach.

- **Better Memory and Concentration**– Having trouble focusing on something? Well then, rosemary might just have the trick for you. Several studies have shown the oil extract coming from rosemary is found to have increased cognitive function and memory for those who have taken it.Components of the herb is said to have a stimulating effect on the nerve roots which enhance memory and concentration.

- **Protects the Nervous System –** Carnosic acid found in rosemary is found to have protective properties for the brain, promoting the health of the nervous system and even fighting off free radical damage that can occur in the brain. Studies have also shown that rosemary protects the brain from aging.

- **Fights Off Cancer –** As you'd expect from one of the best herbs for health, rosemary is found to be quite effective in fighting against cancer. Key components in rosemary were found to have anti-proliferative effects on the excessive white blood cell production found in some forms of leukemia. Adding the anti-inflammatory benefits of rosemary, this herb is quite useful in lowering the risk for cancer.

- **Prevents Macular Degeneration** – Carnosic acid once again comes into play as the key component found in rosemary. As we grow older, the macule of the eyes start to degenerate and sustain damage, leading to blurry vision. In a study conducted at Sanford-Burnham Medical Research Institute, researchers have found out that carnosic acid helps in preventing the macular degeneration process and promote the health of the eyes.

Rosemary is a staple herb at home. It can easily be bought in the store and it's not that hard to grow at home. If you want to revel in all the benefits that rosemary can offer, then it's a smart choice to have this herb around the house all the time. Rosemary comes as chopped or powdered in supermarkets, but if you really want to get all the glorious benefits of this herb, then getting the fresh ones is the best choice.

Chapter 2 - A Fresh Touch of Basil

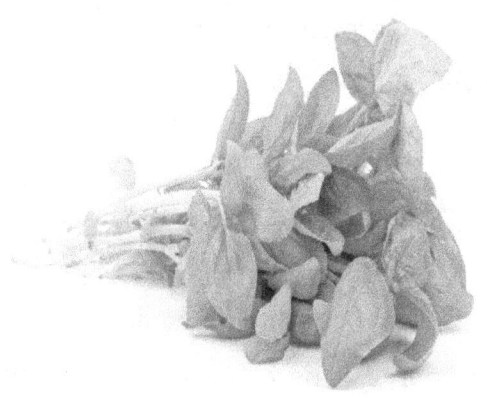

Another common culinary herb, basil or *Ocimumbasilicum* has many other names including St. Joseph's Wort, Thai basil,holy basil, and sweet basil. This herb belongs to the *Lamiaceae* family and possibly native around the regions of India known to be cultivated there for about 5,000 years. Though basil is known to have its Asian origins, it is quite prominent in a wide range of Italian dishes, as well as Southeast Asian dishes like those of Thailand, Vietnam, Taiwan, Cambodia, and Indonesia. Depending on how it's grown, basil may have varying flavor and aroma.

Characteristics

Basil is a versatile herb – some varieties considered as annual while others are considered as perennials. Because of their versatility, basil is known to grow in warmer climates in the tropical regions. One good thing to note about basil is that when the leaves become wilted from a lack of water, you can still save them by watering the herb and putting it under sunlight. Slowly but gradually, the basil leaves can recover their lost green color.

Use of Basil in Cooking

Considered as one of the most common herbs used in cooking, basil is never missing in most Italian and Asian cuisines. A good thing to remember that basil is used as a fresh addition to a dish, it is never cooked. This is because cooking the basil destroys its flavor almost immediately. A complicated herb that's both delicate and versatile, basil increases the flavor, color, and aroma of a dish.

Keeping the basil fresh can be done through a variety of ways. This herb can be put inside a plastic bag and then kept in a refrigerator. Another way is to put basil in a plastic bag and put it in the freezer to keep it for a longer period of time. Just remember to blanch the basil leaves in boiling water to recover its color and freshness. Drying the herbs isn't also advised as it loses its flavor and what remains of the leaves tastes quite different from fresh basil leaves.

Health Benefits of Basil

While most people recognize basil for its wide variety of uses in cooking, it's also known for its various health benefits. To get the most out of basil leaves, you need to consume it fresh as it loses all the vitamins and minerals quickly when cooked. Basil is very rich in Vitamin K, as well as manganese. Other vitamins and minerals found in basil include copper, Vitamin A, Vitamin C, calcium, potassium, iron, and magnesium. The benefits that you can get from basil include the following:

- **Fight Off Stress**–Stress is a normal part of our daily lives, but excessive buildup of stress takes a toll on our health. Basil is found to be effective in fighting off stress as it increases your adrenaline while decreasing the neurotransmitter called serotonin which is known for increasing energy.

- **Relieve Indigestion** – Studies have also shown that drinking tea made from the fresh leaves of basil can help in promoting the health of the digestive tract, expel excessive gas, and prevent constipation. Basil provides relief for those suffering from dyspepsia and abdominal discomfort with its oils promoting a healthy bowel movement.

- **Relieve Headaches** – Basil has a relaxing and soothing effect. When consumed fresh or made into a tea, it can help relieve headaches. Its aromatic scent is known to bring a relaxing sense of rest to the nerves and blood vessels, making it one of the most effective natural remedies for headaches.

- **Natural Detoxifier** – Depending on what you eat, chemicals start to pile up in the liver. Those who often eat fatty foods and junk foods have excessive buildup of waste materials in the liver. What basil does is bind those chemicals in order to help excrete them out of the body which helps in promoting the health of the liver.

- **Lowers the Risk for Breast Cancer** – Studies have shown that tea made from basil leaves have the capability to shrink cancer tumors by limiting the blood supply and halting the metastatic spread of the cancer cells. Be sure to ask your doctor first if you plan to consume basil leaves for lowering the risk for cancer as you may have other conditions that may prevent you from consuming basil.

- **Relieve Anxiety** – Being known for its relaxing effects, basil is also known to relieve mild anxiety. When eaten fresh or turned into a tea, basil can help relieve anxiety through its fragrant aroma and soothing taste. Today, basil even has been used as oils that can be used as fragrance that offer a relaxing effect.

- **Sleep Better** – If you're having trouble sleeping, basil might just be the thing for you. It's rich in melatonin which help in regulating our sleep and wake cycle. This improves sleep and relieves insomnia for those who have trouble sleeping. If you want to adjust your sleeping pattern, then having basil tea or basil oil by the time you sleep can help a lot.

- **Natural Anti-Bacterial** – Basil isn't just about looks and aroma, it's also an effective anti-bacterial that can prevent infections.Because of the amount of bacteria in our environment, there's a high risk in getting an infection without even knowing how you get it. That's why it's important to make use of basil's anti-bacterial capability that's organic and natural. This is because of the volatile oils found in the basil leaves, preventing the growth of various types of bacteria and lowering the risk of infection.

- **Improve Cardiovascular Health** – Basil contains two important things that can help your heart – Vitamin A and Beta-Carotene. These two components help in regulating your blood pressure, promote a healthy heart, and beta-carotene is a powerful anti-oxidant that prevents damage from the harmful free radicals. This lowers the risk of develop heart problems like heart attack, heart failure, and high blood pressure.

Basil is one of the most recognized and widely used herbs in the world. Included in hundreds of European and Asian dishes, the leaves of basil add more flavor, color, and aroma to any cuisine that it's used in. If you want to take advantage of all the health benefits of basil, then go get it at your local supermarket or you can even grow this in your very own garden to make your own supply of this glorious piece of green herb.

Chapter 3–The Rosette Parsley

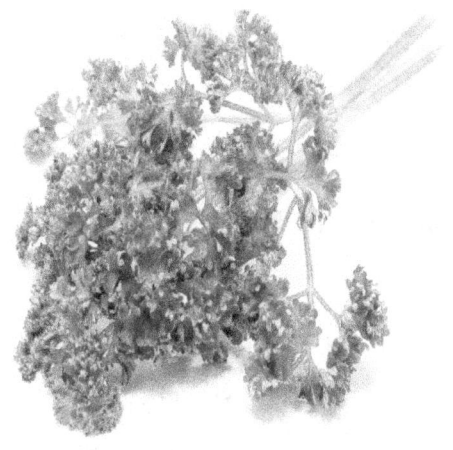

The highest levels of food has never missed the addition of herbs. They add flavor, aroma, and color to the plate. That's why it's essential to have herbs around the kitchen, whether it's your home or it's a five star restaurant. But there's one herb that manages to stand out even more as it is often used in high class restaurants and amazing fine dining dishes. Parsley is probably a name that you've heard of and it's no surprise at how it's used because of its flavor and its benefits towards our health.

Characteristics

Parsley or *Petroselinimcrispum* grows natively around the Mediterranean regions like Tunisia and Italy. It's also found in Europe and it's a common herb and spice that's used in a variety of dishes and in a number of culinary ways. Parsley is a biennial herb that forms a rosette shape of leaves which are used in cooking, fragrances, and even in teas. The taproot of parsley can also be used as a food source that can survive the winter cold and be consumed.

Use of Parsley in Cooking

Parsley is a common herb and spice that adds flavor, color, and aroma to any dish that it's added into. It's mainly used in dishes coming from America, Europe, Brazil, and the Middle East. The leaves of the parsley is also used as a garnish that adds finesse and technique to the dish, most commonly dishes including fish, rice, potatoes, chicken, lamb, and steaks.

Health Benefits of Parsley

Despite its small size, parsley contains a lot of vitamins and minerals that you won't expect from an herb. From Vitamin A to K and with minerals like iron and folate in parsley, there are a lot of benefits that you can get from parsley that promote optimum health and make your dishes a lot healthier aside from being more aromatic, colorful, and flavorsome. Here are some of the health benefits that you can get from eating parsley.

- **Rich in Anti-Oxidants** – Parsley is one of the few herbs that is rich in anti-oxidants. These anti-oxidants help lessen the damage caused by various objects in the environment like pollution, heat, and germs which contain free radicals. Oftentimes, the cells get damaged by free radicals which lead to older and weaker cells. But with anti-oxidants, the growth of newer and healthier cells is boosted.

- **PromotesCardiovascularHealth** – Folic acid and iron are components of parsley which promote the health of the cardiovascular system. These minerals help in promoting the capability of the blood to carry oxygen around the body. These minerals also help in lowering the molecule known as *homocysteine* which increase the risk of getting a heart attack and can even damage the blood vessels when found in excessive amounts.

- **ImproveImmuneSystemFunctio n** – When the body's immune system grows weak, the body become fragile and more prone to develop infections. Vitamin C or ascorbic acid is found in parsley and it helps in promoting the body's immune system. Getting an adequate amount of ascorbic acid is important if y0u want to have a strong immune system.

- **PreventsScurvy** – Severe Vitamin C deficiency can lead to the formation of mouth sores and ulcers which is called *scurvy*. It's not just citrus fruits like lemon or orange that are rich in Vitamin C. Green leafy vegetables also contain a high amount of ascorbic acid and parsley is just one of them.

- **PreventsArthritis** – Studies found that because of the rich Vitamin C content in parsley, arthritis can be prevented as ascorbic acid helps in lowering the risk of developing osteoarthritis – a type of arthritis that occurs with the degenerative process of aging. And because of the anti-inflammatory benefits of parsley, rheumatoid arthritis can also be prevented which is also a type of arthritis though inflammatory in nature.

- **LowerstheRiskofCancer** – Research suggests that parsley has components that slow down the division of cancer cells and cut off the supply of nutrients that go to the cancer cells. Because of the high vitamin and mineral content of parsley, the growth of healthier and younger cells are promoted further.

- **PreventsDiabetes** – In another study, parsley is found to have the capability in lowering blood sugar levels. This helps in lowering the risk of diabetes as blood sugar plays a key role in this health condition. What parsley does is regulate the blood glucose levels, helping decrease the often elevated sugar levels and lower the risk for diabetes to develop.

- **Strengthens the Bones** – A lack of Vitamin K can lead to the degeneration of bones and eventually bone fractures. A rich of source Vitamin K is parsley and even with its small addition, it can help add more Vitamin K to your diet. This will help strengthen your bones and prevent bone-related injuries and diseases like arthritis, fractures, and more.

Four Herbs for Health

Small in nature but big in health benefits, parsley is one formidable opponent when it comes to nutritional value. It can be added in a number of dishes, may it be as a garnish, a design, or a part of the main dish. Parsley is one of the most versatile and easily available herbs that you can get for your kitchen and it helps a lot if you have some at home. If you're still skeptical about parsley, just look at all the health benefits that you can get aside from taste, flavor, color, and aroma.

Chapter 4 - The Power of Cilantro

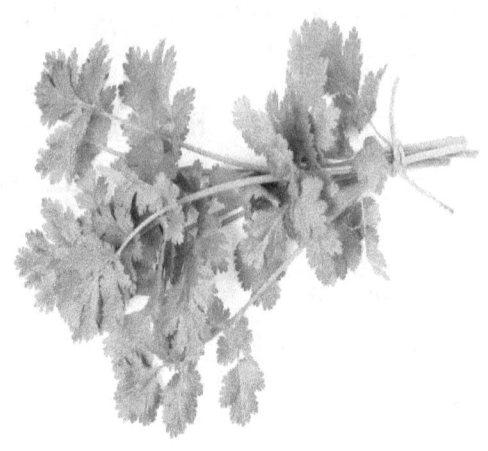

Cilantro is another herb that's common and has become a household name when it comes to common kitchen ingredients. This herb has contrasting features with its delicate and fine green leaves but contains a strong and pungent flavor. While the herb itself is called *cilantro*, the seeds of the herb is called *coriander* which should not be confused with each other. Though these two come from the same plant, cilantro and coriander have very different flavors and uses. But let's focus more on the herb itself with cilantro being the main star of most high end dishes around the world.

Characteristics

Growing natively in southwest Asia, southern Europe, and some parts of Africa, cilantro is a delicate plant that can grow as tall as 20 inches. All the parts of the herb can be eaten and often turned into spices, with its leaves adding color, flavor, and aroma to dishes, while the dried seeds of the herb serves as a strong addition as a flavorsome ingredient. However, there are times when the herb can be eaten alone as it is now used in various oils, teas, and cosmetic products, on top of its culinary uses.

Use of Cilantro in Cooking

Cilantro is a versatile herb that is available all year round. Because of its versatility and its flavor, it can be added in a variety of dishes. Cilantro can be infused within rice, be used in soups, blended into sauces, and used as a spice for meats like chicken and beef. The herb is also used as a frequent garnish to add more color and finesse to various dishes, especially in high-class restaurants.

Health Benefits of Cilantro

Delicate but flavorsome, gentle but strong, and fine yet versatile – these qualities of cilantro make it as a unique type of herb that's used in a variety of ways. Used often in cooking, cilantro is just more than a simple garnish or spice in dishes. It bears powerful benefits towards our health and it's no stranger when it comes to being used as a vital component in various oils, teas, and health products. Here are some of the health benefits of cilantro that you should know.

- Natural Cleansing Agent – Cilantro is unique because of its capability to help detoxify the body from various agents. Various studies have been conducted that cite those who have experienced lead and mercury poisoning reported to have a decreased amount of dizziness, disorientation, and confusion after consuming cilantro. And because it's a natural resource, cilantro doesn't injure the liver and kidneys compared to the commercial chemical detoxifiers.

- Lowers Blood Pressure – Cilantro can help lower the bad cholesterol levels in the blood which also results in lowering the blood pressure. The herb is also rich in potassium which helps control the sodium and potassium ratio in the blood. When there's a high potassium and low sodium ratio in the blood, the blood pressure is kept normal which also helps relieve hypertension.

- Relieves Anxiety – Because of its soothing qualities, cilantro helps in relieve the tension of the muscles. Its relaxing effect allows the nerves to rest and also result in the relief of anxiety. Several people have reported a relief in anxiety after eating cilantro.

- Promotes Adequate Sleep – Due to its relaxing nature, cilantro can also help in promoting a good sleep and wake cycle. The muscles and the nerves are allowed to rest and taking cilantro in your diet helps promote adequate sleep. This is espccially useful for those who are suffering from insomnia and have trouble staying asleep at night.

- Relieves Indigestion – Cilantro helps in promoting a healthy digestive tract. It helps relieve excessive gas and abdominal fullness. This helps in relieving digestive problems like dyspepsia, nausea, and constipation. If you have trouble with your tummy, then a good dose of cilantro might help you. This is also useful for dishes that you'd expect to bloat your stomach, so adding a touch of cilantro might help prevent indigestion.

- Helps Lower Blood Sugar – Because of how easy it is to raise our blood sugar, there comes a point that our blood sugar levels become too high. It's easy to raise blood sugar because of junk food and high caloric foods. Cilantro has a glucose-lowering effect which helps those who have a high blood sugar level like those who have diabetes.

- Anti-Inflammatory Agent – Cilantro is a natural anti-inflammatory agent which helps in relieving swelling and redness for areas that are injured. Compared to the anti-inflammatory drugs that you can buy commercially, cilantro is organic and natural, so you don't have to worry about nasty side effects like taking its toll on your liver and kidneys.

- Organic Anti-Oxidant – This herb is a powerful anti-oxidant which helps in fighting off damage caused by free radicals. These free radicals can be found in a lot of things like dust, pollution, heat, and germs. This helps in promoting the health of the cells by encouraging the growth of newer and healthier cells.

- Promotes Smoother and Healthier Skin – Cilantro is one of the few herbs that is used in various skin care products. This is because cilantro promotes the healthy growth of cells, thus promoting a healthier growth of the skin. Cilantro helps in shaving off the old and dying cells of the skin, making room for newer skin cells.

There are certainly a lot more benefits that cilantro brings to the table. It has a unique flavor, aroma, and uses just like the other herbs. But it certainly takes its place as being one of the most valuable and useful herbs that you can have.

Conclusion

Herbs are one of the staple and most basic ingredients around the kitchen. They can easily be added to any dish to add more flavor, color, and aroma. However, it isn't just about the culinary use of herbs, but it's also about the various health benefits that these herbs can bring. But the thing about herbs is that they often go ignored and overlooked as most people opt to the more robust and easiest approach in cooking.

After knowing the various health benefits of the most essential herbs in the world, cooking has now changed for you and your family. Herbs come as cheap and easily accessible. If you want to make use of all the benefits that these herbs can bring, why not head to your nearest supermarket and get your favorite herb. If not, then why not grow your very own herbs in your own garden as well?

www.ingramcontent.com/pod-product-compliance
Lightning Source LLC
Chambersburg PA
CBHW071252280526
45788CB00004B/1679